What Next, After Cholelithiasis?

Rowena Kong

2020

First Printing: 2020

ISBN: 9798634411422

Gallbladder disease commonly affects the general population of Western developed nations and the standard surgical treatment of laparoscopic cholecystectomy normally follows severe cases of this condition. However, the negative health and life quality consequences of this standard line of treatment are lesser-known and stand the chance of being taken lightly by healthcare professionals. Complications include bile duct injury, dropped gallstones and a second open invasive surgery, of which could be life-threatening for some rare cases. It is therefore, necessary to highlight the limitations of such a procedure and the need for improvement and widening of the range of treatment options for vulnerable members of the patient population. Additionally, here is a brief overview introduction of a new procedure called endoscopic ultrasound-guided gallbladder drainage with promising success rates that can be a potentially feasible alternative to traditional surgical procedures to offer gallbladder disease patients.

Introduction

At present, there is a very limited non-surgical options for the management and removal of gallstones, a condition which affects a considerable part of the population in developed nations. However, cases abound where surgery is not an option for high-risk patients and the possibility of long-term undesirable consequences arising from the removal is not unlikely. No doubt, the surgical removal of gallbladder is the main treatment option for the management of gallbladder disease or acute and chronic cholecystitis, a condition due to the formation of gallstones in the gallbladder. The surgical procedure of laparoscopic cholecystectomy is now frequently performed in addition to the traditional and more invasive open cholecystectomy. However, this new procedure which has evolved from open cholecystectomy is not completely without risks and complications. On the other hand, patients may refuse such standard surgical treatment due to the daunting prospect of permanently losing an organ that has significant described functions necessary for a wholesome digestive health. Although it is assumed that avoidance of negative and progressive pathophysiological outcome based on immediate and short-term basis of consideration necessitates the removal of a gallbladder, this generally accepted approach may mask compromised and unpredictable normal healthy functioning of the digestive tract on the long-term.

1   Surgical risks and potential complications

Occurrences of bile duct injury and dropped gallstones can result from the increasingly common procedure of laparoscopic cholecystectomy.[1, 2, 3] Bile duct injury carries a high risk of morbidity and mortality and may require a follow-up reconstruction surgical procedure for the majority of patients who encounter such complication.[4] In certain cases, this second reconstruction surgery for bile duct injury deemed necessary is associated with increased mortality. Nonetheless, one national survey study reported that such reconstruction surgery was necessary for 64% of all major bile duct injuries. [5] At other times, there was also a high risk of up to 30% of converting a laparoscopic cholecystectomy procedure into more invasive open cholecystectomy for patients who are above 50 years of age.[6] Unfortunately, the risk of developing bile duct injury actually increases with laparoscopic cholecystectomy more than traditional open cholecystectomy.[7] Therefore, the new benefit comes at a cost of higher risk for a particular life-threatening surgical complication. Despite increasing experience with cholecystectomy, one study reported a 0.23% rate of occurrence of bile duct injury which required follow-up surgical intervention as well as an association with 9.84% 30-day morbidity rate that included conditions such as intestinal disorders, infectious and shock complications.[8] As for long-term mortality associated with bile duct injury that required surgical intervention, another study reported a high rate of 20.8%.[9]

2   Discussion

Unlike bile duct injury, which may have a low rate of occurrence in spite of its life-threatening consequences, a more common complication of cholecystectomy is dropped gallstones which can be retained in the body. [10] However, what is more disheartening about such outcome on asymptomatic patients is that such complication may go undetected until fistula and abscess in the gastrointestinal tract are discovered only months or years post-surgery. Further infection and serious morbidities may result from such retainment even though the post-procedural removal of dropped gallstones are often challenging for the surgeon.[11, 12]

Another negative outcome associated with laparoscopic cholecystectomy is a high risk of up to 30% of procedure conversion to more invasive open cholecystectomy for patients who are above 50 years of age. [6] With regards to surgical intervention required for the previously mentioned complication of bile duct injury for laparoscopic cholecystectomy, there was one certain case of a patient who needed a liver transplant at about 4 years after having undergone such procedure.[9] Therefore, the limited number of recent long-term follow-up studies which comprehensively assessed related negative impact on the quality of life of patients who have undergone such surgeries may overestimate the feasibility of such invasive procedures. [13] There can be both short-term and long-term negative consequences on the health and life of patients which arise from possible complications of laparoscopic cholecystectomy. Nevertheless, the goal of such surgery should be to provide improvement from traditional open surgery and lasting benefit(s) as much as possible while achieving minimal level of invasiveness and the lowest rate of complications. However, with the risk of serious bile duct injury, dropped gallstones and conversion to open cholecystectomy, this may suggest the need for development of less invasive and non-surgical procedures for the treatment of gallbladder disease that can offer the promise of better long-term quality of life for patients who wish to keep their gallbladder and those who are advanced in age. It therefore cannot be denied that surgical outcomes can have lasting negative impact on the quality of life of patients which may not have immediate remedial options. There are also not many long-term follow-up studies of patients which comprehensively assess related negative impact on the quality of life of those who have undergone surgery, which may overestimate the feasibility of such invasive procedures. [13]

Despite the limitations and possible detrimental outcomes of surgical treatment of gallstone disease, one notable advancement in this area is the new technique called endoscopic ultrasound-guided gallbladder drainage or more often known as endoscopic ultrasound-guided transmural drainage. [14, 15] This procedure is, as its name suggests, one that makes use of an endoscope with the ability to visualize the internal organs through ultrasound imaging that will guide its entry and pathway into the stomach or duodenum and finally reaches the gallbladder. The gallstones will be drained using stents which can be made from more than one type of choice material, e.g. plastic or metal, out of the gallbladder into the gastrointestinal tract using other devices. Each type of stent material has its own advantages over the other, e.g. different success rates and the number of post-procedural adverse events.[16, 17]

In general, both the technical and clinical success rates of this new procedure are over 90%, making it a positive and appealing choice for high-risk and elderly patients who cannot undergo surgery. However, there remains a question whether this option can be extended to those who are fit for surgery but would like to keep their gallbladder organ with them. Presently, there is limited documentation on the comparison of long-term outcome between laparoscopic cholecystectomy (and related surgical treatments) and endoscopic ultrasound-guided gallbladder drainage as the latter is still a young procedure that is yet to be widely available. However, the recurrence rate of cholecystitis, which is the inflammation of the gallbladder due to the presence of gallstones that was consequently resolved after this gallbladder drainage procedure, is less than 4%, according to Law and Baron [15]. Furthermore, earlier higher risk of adverse events associated with the use of plastic stents has been lowered with current preference for self-expandable metal stents and lumen-apposing metal stents. A recent Food and Drug Administration-approved version of lumen-apposing metal stent with a catheter tip can be employed without a guidewire in certain patients, thereby minimising related complications. A first successful case of utilizing lumen-apposing metal stent with guidewire has been performed on an elderly patient who had previously undergone partial gastrectomy and deemed unfit for laparoscopic cholecystectomy as well as percutaneous transhepatic gallbladder drainage.[18] In this specific case, there was no record of adverse event both during the procedure and follow-up with the patient at 3 months.

Conclusion

There seem to be considerable positive outcomes with endoscopic ultrasound-guided gallbladder drainage, despite the cases of bleeding during the performance of the procedure that have been documented. [19] It should also be noted that this could be done on high-risk patients who may be on anticoagulant medications and/or having comorbid health conditions which already carry an underlying risk of bleeding prior to the procedure. Although multiple large gallstones have been seen removed through this method, it is wondered whether the size and number of stones contained in the gallbladder positively correlate with the level of risk of probable complications that could arise and future studies should investigate this variable aspect and outcome(s) of the procedure. It is also reasonable to assume that lumen-apposing metal stents with upgrade(s) in functional features and flexibility, such as electrocautery-enhanced,[18] would gain appreciation and popularity in impending challenging case attempts. With increasing elderly populations in a number of regions in the world, it could be anticipated that patient candidates for traditional and standard cholecystectomy would fall into unsuitable older age groups that demand more catered procedure options. The advances in endoscopic ultrasound guided gallbladder drainage from the early percutaneous transhepatic method to transpapillary and finally, transmural type of access with the latest lumen-apposing metal stents, speak for its fast-evolving development in broadening and improving treatment reach and access to otherwise unfit patient groups. Studies have documented similar technical and clinical success rates and lower rates of long-term adverse event outcomes and **recurrent acute cholecystitis between endoscopic ultrasound guided** gallbladder drainage and percutaneous transhepatic cholecystostomy.[20] On the other hand, a decreased occurrence of recurrent cholecystitis may not completely signify a lack of gallstone reformation or development. A follow-up with the patient to the procedure could additionally determine this occurrence in order to comprehensively compare such non-surgical endoscopic and standard surgical outcomes. The rate and duration of gallstone reformation, of which the etiology also remains uncertain and highly variable among patient populations, with such a comparison could assist in scrutinising the long-standing rationale behind the choice in decision to urgently proceed with laparoscopic cholecystectomy during acute stages of patient cases. While the long-term comparison of the above aspect variables in determining the competing feasibility between gallbladder drainage and laparoscopic cholecystectomy is still limited, the latter's more invasive technique which carries a longer and more diverse list of potential risks and complications and uncertain compromised normal digestive tract functioning and quality of life is worth a consideration for a perspective revision of its gold standard treatment approach status. Ultimately, a random trial design of study between these two procedures with careful selection of diverse groups of patient subjects and well-matched demographics would be necessary to assess both the short-term and long-term desirability in terms of treatment approach, prognosis and quality of life outcomes. It is therefore suggested that surgical risks, in spite of how minimal and below chance of occurrence they may be, should not be ignored and taken less heed of, because each patient case should be treated as unique as an autonomous individual with personal history and needs that vary from the rest. Surgical professionals must be prepared at all times to address and handle untimely and unanticipated procedural complications.

References

1. Moore DE, Feurer ID, Holzman MD, Wudel LJ, Strickland C, Gorden DL, Chari R, Wright JK, Pinson CW. Long-term detrimental effect of bile duct injury on health-related quality of life. Archives of Surgery. 2004 May 5;139(5):476-82.

2. Ragozzino A, Puglia M, Romano F, Imbriaco M. Intra-Hepatic spillage of gallstones as a late complication of laparoscopic cholecystectomy: MR imaging findings. Polish journal of radiology. 2016;81:322.

3. Schreuder AM, Booij KA, de Reuver PR, van Delden OM, van Lienden KP, Besselink MG, Busch OR, Gouma DJ, Rauws EA, van Gulik TM. Percutaneous-endoscopic rendezvous procedure for the management of bile duct injuries after cholecystectomy: short-and long-term outcomes. Endoscopy. 2018 Jun;50(06):577-87.

4. Worth PJ, Kaur T, Diggs BS, Sheppard BC, Hunter JG, Dolan JP. Major bile duct injury requiring operative reconstruction after laparoscopic cholecystectomy: a follow-on study. Surgical endoscopy. 2016 May 1;30(5):1839-46.

5. Archer SB, Brown DW, Smith CD, Branum GD, Hunter JG. Bile duct injury during laparoscopic cholecystectomy: results of a national survey. Annals of surgery. 2001 Oct;234(4):549.

6. *Cholecystectomy: Surgical removal of the gallbladder* [Internet]. Chicago: American College of Surgeons; 2018 [cited 2019 Sept 11]. Available from: https://www.facs.org/~/media/files/education/patient%20ed/cholesys.ashx

7. Nuzzo G, Giuliante F, Giovannini I, Ardito F, D'Acapito F, Vellone M, Murazio M, Capelli G. Bile duct injury during laparoscopic cholecystectomy: results of an Italian national survey on 56 591 cholecystectomies. Archives of Surgery. 2005 Oct 1;140(10):986-92.

8. Barrett M, Asbun HJ, Chien HL, Brunt LM, Telem DA. Bile duct injury and morbidity following cholecystectomy: a need for improvement. Surgical endoscopy. 2018 Apr 1;32(4):1683-8.

9. Halbert C, Altieri MS, Yang J, Meng Z, Chen H, Talamini M, Pryor A, Parikh P, Telem DA. Long-term outcomes of patients with common bile duct injury

following laparoscopic cholecystectomy. Surgical endoscopy. 2016 Oct 1;30(10):4294-9.

10. Binagi S, Keune J, Awad M. Immediate postoperative pain: an atypical presentation of dropped gallstones after laparoscopic cholecystectomy. Case reports in surgery. 2015;2015.

11. Nooghabi AJ, Hassanpour M, Jangjoo A. Consequences of lost gallstones during laparoscopic cholecystectomy: a review article. Surgical Laparoscopy Endoscopy & Percutaneous Techniques. 2016 Jun 1;26(3):183-92.

12. Thomson B, Kawa B, Rabone A, Abdul-Aal Y, Hasan F, Ignotus P, Shaw A. Ultrasound-guided percutaneous retrieval of a dropped gallstone following laparoscopic cholecystectomy. BJR| case reports. 2018 Apr;4(3):20180002.

13. Booij KA, de Reuver PR, van Dieren S, van Delden OM, Rauws EA, Busch OR, van Gulik TM, Gouma DJ. Long-term impact of bile duct injury on morbidity, mortality, quality of life, and work related limitations. Annals of surgery. 2018 Jul 1;268(1):143-50.

14. Peñas-Herrero I, de la Serna-Higuera C, Perez-Miranda M. Endoscopic ultrasound-guided gallbladder drainage for the management of acute cholecystitis (with video). Journal of Hepato-Biliary-Pancreatic Sciences. 2015 Jan 1;22(1):35-43.

15. Law R, Baron TH. Endoscopic Ultrasound-Guided Gallbladder Drainage. Gastrointestinal endoscopy clinics of North America. 2018 Apr;28(2):187-95.

16. Anderloni A, Buda A, Vieceli F, Khashab MA, Hassan C, Repici A. Endoscopic ultrasound-guided transmural stenting for gallbladder drainage in high-risk patients with acute cholecystitis: a systematic review and pooled analysis. Surgical endoscopy. 2016 Dec 1;30(12):5200-8.

17. Teoh AY, Serna C, Penas I, Chong CC, Perez-Miranda M, Ng EK, Lau JY. Endoscopic ultrasound-guided gallbladder drainage reduces adverse events compared with percutaneous cholecystostomy in patients who are unfit for cholecystectomy. Endoscopy. 2017 Feb;49(02):130-8.

18. Anderloni A, Fugazza A, Maroni L, Troncone E, Milani O, Cappello A, Alkandari A, Repici A. Endoscopic ultrasound-guided gallbladder drainage by transduodenal

lumen-apposing metal stent in a patient with Roux-en-Y reconstruction. Annals of gastroenterology. 2019 Sep;32(5):522.

19. Saumoy M, Kahaleh M. Safety and complications of interventional endoscopic ultrasound. Clinical endoscopy. 2018 May;51(3):235.

20. Chan JH, Teoh AY. Current status of endoscopic gallbladder drainage. Clinical endoscopy. 2018 Mar;51(2):150.

www.ingramcontent.com/pod-product-compliance
Lightning Source LLC
Chambersburg PA
CBHW031513210526
45463CB00008B/3219